I0415040

Essential Oils for Allergies

Essential Oil Recipes for
Allergies
for Diffusers, Roller Bottles, Inhalers & more.

Rica V. Gadi

Copyright © 2019 by The Oil Natural Empress

All rights reserved. This book or any portion thereof may not be reproduced or used in any manner whatsoever without the express written permission of the publisher except for the use of brief quotations in a book review.

Printed in the United States of America

First Printing, 2019

ISBN: 9781086035230

http://eorecipes.net

DISCLAIMER: This document is a compilation of recipes used successfully by EO enthusiasts who use only high-quality, therapeutic-grade essential oils as determined by many factors including growth, growth location, harvesting process, distillation method used, etc. Please be advised that not all essential oils are created equally, and not all essential oils are suitable for topical use or ingestion. Please do your research before choosing the brand(s) of essential oils you decide to use as well as the supplies you use. Always follow label directions on the essential oil bottles.

All the recipes in this book have been inspired by essential oil believers. However, we are not medical practitioners and cannot diagnose, treat or prescribe treatment for any health condition or disease. Just a precaution, before using any alternative medicine, natural supplements, or vitamins, you should always discuss the products you are using or intend to use with your doctor, especially if you are pregnant, trying to get pregnant or nursing.

All information contained within this book is for reference purposes only, and is not intended to substitute for advice given by a pharmacist, physician or other licensed health-care professional. As such, the author is not responsible for any loss, claim or damage arising from the use of the essential oil recipes contained herein.

This book is dedicated to all the strong people who are taking responsibility for your own well being and doing something to be better.

All my heartfelt gratitude to the following people: my mom Ruby Jane, you have made me everything I am today; my dad Nestor-- my eternal, my angel, and the source of my perseverance; Mommyling, my spiritual guide ; Ria & Joe, the true witnesses of my transformation and my foundation pillars; Ellie Jane, the sparkle of our eyes;

Juan, thanks for always encouraging me to push harder - you are my ONE; Rocco & Radha, my reason for everything.

The Love of my family and friends is the fountain of inspiration that never runs dry. Thank you for constantly inspiring me, motivating me, and loving me unconditionally.

This book will never be complete without the help of my trusted and talented friends the #NOWsuperstars and my #oilbularya friends

Blending Essential Oils to use for a very specific reason has become very popular in recent years. There are several reasons why this is so. Blending EOs is basically about inhaling - as it has been proven that aromas have the ability to trigger feelings, emotions and personal memories.

With this in mind, it is obvious that everyone is unique when it comes to what triggers your senses. It all boils down to personal preference for the aroma to trigger what you want to unleash. Everyone is different and we all connect to the aroma differently, so what might work for one might not work for another person.

Of course, we also want the blend we personalize to be therapeutic. This is the best reason why to blend essential oils. We want the blend we create to help us with a very specific emotion or physical condition. As much as smelling good is important in a blend, it is more important that we blend oils that are not only pleasing to the smell but also produces the therapeutic effect we are after.

Then you have to think about contraindications. Making sure the blend you create is safe to use.

I suggest that before blending find out if the oils you are using is safe for a condition you may have example, if you are pregnant, or have specific allergies. Consult your physician prior to moving forward.

The recipes I have in this book is a compilation of what has proven to work and favored by hundreds of EO enthusiasts. It takes out the guesswork to get you started.

Again, we urge you to read the recipes and make sure that this is safe for you to try.

The book is very specific to a physical and emotional condition. There are several recipes here because you might want to rotate and you may like one and not the other. There is also a variety of applications. Some of us prefer to diffuse, some to make roller bottles, and others to create inhalers and sprays.

I hope you enjoy this compilation, feel free to use the notes section and jot down your fave blends. There is a wonderful world of EO blending - this is just the beginning.

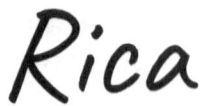

A person having an allergy means that they have a hypersensitivity or intolerance to substances that are not typically harmful to other people. This is unique to an individual's immune system and that means that different individuals have different types of allergies. There are some that have been blessed without allergies but for a lot of people, allergies are hereditary and have been passed from generation to generation. Allergens come in different forms like food or other materials like pollen, fur or dust.

Allergies can happen when an individual comes into contact with an allergen. When an allergic reaction happens, a lot of symptoms can take place. There are different body parts that can be affected by the symptoms caused by an allergic reaction. The most common body parts that can be affected are the nose, eyes, and throat. Some people experience swelling of the sinus which can cause severe sneezing, redness of the eyes or a sore throat when faced with an allergic reaction. The lungs can also be affected, wherein breathing becomes difficult due to swelling in passages to the lungs. Allergic reactions can be in the form of an upset stomach as well which is common for people with food allergies. Allergic reactions can also cause skin irritations, inflammation, and redness.

It is best to seek the help of a doctor at the onset of an allergy in order to immediately find a remedy for it and to know the specific allergen that caused the reaction. Some people may be aware of the allergies they have starting from when they are children and in these cases, they would already know what medication to use to reduce the reactions.

Home remedies that can help reduce and soothe symptoms that are caused by allergies can be made with essential oils. Although there are different types of allergies, there are specific essential oils that can help soothe the symptoms of any type of allergies. Essential oils like eucalyptus can help inflammatory reactions like on the nose and skin. The cooling sensation of eucalyptus oils can reduce congestion and provide relief. Ginger oil is an expectorant and can help in allergies caused by dust and dirt that also affects the lungs. These examples of essential oils can help soothe allergies but it is also crucial to be aware that essential oils can also be allergens that can cause an allergic reaction depending on the person. It is best to seek advice from a doctor before taking this home remedy.

Table of Contents

Best Essential Oils for Allergies

You may experience seasonal allergies in late winter or spring or even in late summer and fall. Allergies may occur occasionally as a plant you're allergic to blooms. Or, you may experience around-the-clock allergies during specific seasonal months.

Essential oils may be used as an alternative or complementary treatment for allergy symptoms. They're derived from plants and can be used in a variety of ways. There are a lot of Popular ways to use essential oils like diffusing them into the air, using them in the bath and spa products, applying them to the skin when diluted, spraying them into the air or breathing them in directly from the container

Breathing in the oils' scents is known as aromatherapy. This practice stimulates your body through your sense of smell. What you smell can affect other parts of your body.Just like with aromatherapy, applying the oils to your body results in them entering your bloodstream. You should always dilute the essential oils before using them on your skin.A carrier oil, such as sweet almond oil or olive oil, can work well for this purpose. You usually mix about 5 drops of the essential oil to 1 ounce of carrier oil.

There isn't a great deal of research to support the use of essential oils, but more is coming out all the time. If done with care, aromatherapy with essential oils might benefit you.If you'd like to incorporate essential oils into your life to relieve allergy symptoms, here are a few you might want to try.

1. Lavender

Lavender is a popular essential oil because of its many benefits.It may help soothe your symptoms during allergy season thanks to its ability to calm and reduce inflammation. One study concluded that the essential oil prevents allergic inflammation as well as the enlargement of mucous cells.Try using lavender in a diffuser for aromatherapy or dilute it in a carrier oil and soak in a bath with a bit added.

2. Blend of sandalwood, frankincense, and Ravensara oil

One study used a blend of sandalwood, frankincense, and Ravensara oils to treat perennial allergic rhinitis. Study participants reported improvement with their blocked nasal passages, runny and itchy noses, and sneezing.This suggests that this blend of essential oils can help with perceived symptoms, quality of life related to allergies, and better sleep.To use these blended oils, mix with a carrier oil (such as sweet almond oil) and apply to the skin. They can also be diffused into the air.

3. Peppermint

Peppermint essential oil is known to reduce inflammationTrusted Source. You'll be able to breathe easier by diffusing the oil or even applying it on your skin after it's diluted with a carrier oil.Combining peppermint with lavender and lemon oils creates an effective and soothing allergy relief combination as well. However, be aware that combined oils can increase your chances of having an allergic reaction. If you apply citrus oils, you will be sun-sensitive.

4. Lemon

Citrus-scented essential oils are often used in aromatherapy to boost alertness and energy. Lemon essential oil can also help clear your sinuses and reduce congestion, common symptoms of seasonal allergies.Be careful exposing your skin to sunlight or tanning beds if you're using lemon or any citrus-scented oils. Try diffusing the oil to lift your mood or diluting and applying it to your skin to help with allergy symptoms.

5. Eucalyptus

Eucalyptus oil is known as an anti-inflammatory and may help you with your congestion. The cooling sensation you experience while breathing it in may also help you feel relief as you deal with and treat seasonal allergies.Researchers are beginning to understand how using eucalyptus aromatherapy reduces inflammation. This could lead to reducing allergic symptoms.

Try diffusing eucalyptus into the air or breathing it in from the bottle to provide you with comfort.

Despite showing anti-inflammatory properties, eucalyptus can also trigger allergies in some people.

6. Tea Tree Oil

Tea tree oil is an inexpensive oil. While a beneficial addition to your allergy prevention and treatment shelf, there are more restrictions with this essential oil. Tea tree oil should never be ingested; it is a topical remedy only. You should also avoid using tea tree oil along with lavender oil on boys who have not yet reached puberty. This may cause abnormal hormone effects.

Because this is a topical use oil, most benefits are in relation to skin irritations. Tea tree oil reduces the redness and the circumference of an allergic reaction. Adding the oil to hair conditioner will not only kill and repel lice and their eggs, but it will also kill mites found on eyelashes and beards that can cause allergic irritations and rashes. It is also suggested that adding tea tree oil to body wash can soothe irritations from bed bugs.

The Blending Process

These EOs are categorized by aromas, and EOs from the same group usually blend fantastically together.

- Floral – Lavender, Geranium, Jasmine
- Woodsy – Pine, Cedarwood
- Earthy – Vetiver, Patchouli
- Herbaceous – Marjoram, Rosemary, Basil
- Minty – Peppermint, Spearmint, Wintergreen
- Medicinal – Eucalyptus, Frankincense, Melaleuca
- Spicy – Pepper, Clove, Cinnamon
- Oriental – Ginger, Patchouli
- Citrus – Wild Orange, Lemon, Lime

Select oils that will give you with the health benefits you are looking to remedy. For increased energy choose: Grapefruit, Lemon, Orange, or Citrus. For Calming and Relaxation choose: Lavender, Cedarwood, or Chamomile. You are encouraged to experiment and play with your oils to see which blends work for you.

TIPS:

- Combine Floral EOs with Woodsy, Spicy and Citrus aromas
- Minty EOs with Woodsy, Earthy, Herbaceous and Citrus aromas
- Earthy EOs with Woodsy and Minty aromas
- Citrus EOs with Floral, Woodsy, Minty, Spicy and Oriental aromas

Diffuse

Diffusing Essential Oils is the safest method to enjoy Essential Oils without the risk of an allergic reaction.

Diffusing Essential Oils
Some Tidbits You Need To Know

Our sense of smell is one of our most powerful senses, and as you have noticed in your own experience that some scents affect your more positively in your minds than others. The body contains over 1,000 receptors for smell—way more receptors than for any of our other senses.

Diffusion Essential Oils means the process vaporizes oils into the air by releasing tiny amounts into the air. Inhalation is totally safe and is super low risk. Chances of any EO rising to dangerous levels while diffusion is slim to none.

Diffusing Essential Oils around newborns, babies, young children, pregnant or nursing women, and pets should be done with caution. Read up on safety.

It is advisable that Diffusing Essential Oils for only about 15-30 minutes at a time to be most effective. NEVER leave your diffuser on overnight. Make sure your diffuser is filled with the right amount of water and you understand the operating directions.

While diffusing essential oils, be sure that your space has great ventilation. Crack a window open if the scent becomes strong.

Never add Carrier Oils to your diffuser. This may cause your diffuser to malfunction. Clean your diffuser at least 3 times a week with warm water and natural soap to ensure the diffuser is well maintained and bacteria and mold does not accumulate.

Diffusing Essential Oils
Basic Guidelines

Just a few things you need to know and prepare before getting started Diffusing Essential Oils.

Things you need:
Ultrasonic Oil Diffuser
Essential Oils
Water

Just follow the number of drops in the recipe, drop on to an oil diffuser and fill the rest with water.

All diffusers are different and will have its own water minimum and maximum level. Read the diffuser instruction before use.

Ideally, it is best to diffuse for 15-30 minutes and turn off the diffuser. The effect should be good for at least 2-3 hours. Turn your diffuser back on after 3 hours to reinforce oil diffusing effects.

It is not advisable to use EO in humidifiers.

These are not made to release EOS

Diffuser Recipes

Here's a thought for you:

You may be wondering how aroma can simply eliminate symptoms. There's a simple answer to this : Aroma is simply a by-product of diffusing. It's the added benefit but in reality the real benefit comes from the air we breathe and how the body easily absorbs the essential oils released into the air. It works 2 ways, not only does it improve the air quality you breath by disinfecting and eliminating pollutants it also allows your glands to absorb the healing elements of the EOs released in the air molecules,

So here are a few recipes that can help you manage symptoms and actual issues regarding the matter :

3 Drops Peppermint
3 Drops Lavender
3 Drops Lemon

----

3 Drops Peppermint
3 Drops Lemon
3 Drops Lavender

----

2 Lavender
2 Lemon
2 Peppermint (+ 2 Melaleuca, optional)

----

5 Drops Lavender
3 Drops Vetiver
2 Drops Ylang Ylang

----

3 Drops Peppermint
2 Drops Eucalyptus
2 Drops Tea Tree
1 Drop Lemon

----

3 Drops Peppermint
3 Drops Lemon
3 Drops Eucalyptus

----

3 Drops Tea Tree
2 Drops Lavender
2 Drops Peppermint

----

4 Drops Lavender
4 Drops Peppermint
2 Drops Frankincense
2 Drops Basil

----

3 Drops Eucalyptus
3 Drops Peppermint
3 Drops Rosemary

----

1 Drop Lemongrass
1 Drop Melaleuca
1 Drop Thyme
1 Drop Eucalyptus
1 Drop Rosemary
----

3 drops Lavender
3 drops Peppermint
3 drops Lemon
----

2 drops Peppermint
2 drops Lemon
2 drops Lavender
2 drops Chamomile
----

2 drops Balsam Fir
3 drops Peppermint
2 drops Bay Leaf
1 drops Red Thyme

----

2 drops Eucalyptus
2 drops Peppermint
2 drops Helichrysum
2 drops Lemon

----

3 drops Helichrysum
2 drops Rosemary
2 drops Lavender
2 drops Basil

----

3 drops Tea Tree
2 drops Balsam Fir
2 drops Chamomile
1 drop Bay Leaf

Roll

Essential Oil Roller Bottles is the easiest method to enjoy Essential Oils Anywhere and Whenever.

Blending Essential Oils in a Roller Bottle
Some Tidbits You Need To Know

Essential Oils are usually super concentrated and too hard to measure how much to actually put straight from the bottle.

Roller bottles are a way that you are able to create blends ready to use with the right dilution. It allows your EO to last longer.

It also makes it easier to apply exactly where you want to target without getting it all over the place.

It is handy and easy to carry in your purse, ready to use at any time you want to.

I like to apply EOs at the bottom of the feet for many reasons. Our feet have bigger pores than any other skin in our bodies. this means that they are able to suck in the therapeutic compounds in our blend into the bloodstream faster than any other parts of the body. Imagine comparing a normal straw to an oversized straw and how much more you can suck in with the latter. This is how the soles of our feet is compared to the rest of the skin in our bodies.

The skin on our feet is also less sensitive and is designed to withstand some abuse. The risk of having an irritation from EOS is less likely to happen when applied on the feet.

The feet don't have the glands that act as a barrier. Sebaceous glands are glands in our skin that produces an oily substance called Sebum, for the purpose of lubricating and waterproofing the skin. Since this is oil and if you put oil on top of oil, it can act as a barrier or it may slow down penetration.

The feet and palms of our hands are the only skin that don't have these, so it is ideal to apply Essential Oils to the feet for maximum penetration.

Now, it would be hard to apply oils directly and very messy, right? Roller bottles make it super easy and convenient to roll the EOs at the bottom of our feet.

Carrier Oils Info

Carrier oils are vegetable-based oils with their own healing properties that dilute essential oils used to help carry the EOs into the skin.

Essential oils are highly concentrated and could evaporate very quickly. The carrier oil is mixed with the essential oil so it could penetrate the skin before it actually evaporates. Although EOs are oils, it is actually not that oily. When mixed with a carrier oil, it allows you to have more of the essential oil into your skin without wasting EOS to evaporate, making the healing properties of the EO strong and more effective.

There are also Essential oils that are too strong to apply directly to the skin and may cause damage, so it is important to dilute them with a carrier oil.

Never add Carrier Oils to your diffuser. This may cause your diffuser to malfunction. Clean your diffuser at least 3 times a week with warm water and natural soap to ensure the diffuser is well maintained and bacteria and mold does not accumulate.

Carrier Oils

There are a lot of different carrier oils that you can use with EOs to dilute them in a roller bottle.

To name a few :

Almond Oil - moisturizing and stays liquid at room temperature. Do not use if you are allergic to nuts.

Apricot Kernel Oil - moisturizing and suitable for sensitive skin or kids. It is super gentle on the skin.

Avocado Oil - moisturizing and suitable for sensitive and damaged skin. Perfect for skin problems.Can be mixed with other carrier oils

Castor Oil - with antibacterial, antiviral and antifungal properties, use topically to eliminate pain and relieve skin irritation.

Coconut Oil - its antibacterial, antiviral and antifungal properties it is the best and most versatile for skin care. The skin absorbs this very quickly. It solidifies in room temp and may still have a slight coconut oil aroma in it - but you can get fractionated coconut oil to eliminate the 2 challenges above.

Grapeseed Oil - not just for cooking but also great for topical application on the skin.

Jojoba Oil - one of my faves for skin care blends. This oil is the closest to our natural oil our skin produces to it is absorbed easily without being oily. Also amazing for massage oil blends.

Olive Oil - this is the oil for herb type oils. mostly used for cooking but can also be applied to the skin but would need to be blended with a carrier oil that is mild and absorb well with the skin.

Rosehip Seed Oil - super good for deep moisturizing or skin irritations. This oil has a high content of antioxidants and helps remedy dry, scarred and wounded skin.

Recommended Roller Bottle Dilution Guide

RECOMMENDED ROLL-ON BOTTLE DILUTION AMOUNTS

5 ml (1/6 oz.) Roll-on Bottle = ~100 drops (1tsp.)
10 ml (1/3 oz.) Roll-on Bottle = ~200 drops (2 tsp.)
30 ml. (1 oz.) Roll-on Bottle = ~600 drops (6 tsp.)

Roll-on Size	5 ml	10 ml	30 ml	Add EO drops to roll-on, then fill with carrier oil.	
Essential Oil Drops	1	2	6	1%	Dilution Percentage
	2	4	12	2%	
	3	6	18	3%	
	5	10	30	5%	
	10	20	60	10%	
	20	40	120	20%	
	25	50	150	25%	
	50	100	300	50%	

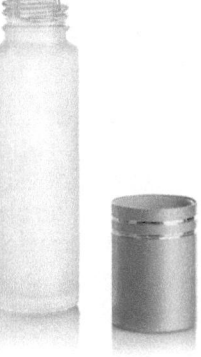

General Guidelines:
Birth to 12 months = .3-.5% dilution
1-5 years = 1.5-3% dilution
6-11 years = 1.5-5% dilution
12-17 years = 1.5-20% dilution
18 years and older = 1.5% dilution-Neat (no dilution)
Elderly or Sensitive Skin = 1-3% dilution
Daily Use = 2-5% dilution
Short Term Use = 10-25% dilution
Local Skin or Systemic Issues = 50% dilution-Neat

These are general guidelines suggestions--not absolute rules--based on traditional aromatheraphy practice.
(Kurt Schnaubelt PhD, Valerie Worwood, Robert Tisserand)

Dilution Basics:

How much you dilute your EO depends on different factors such as weight, sensitivity, health conditions, EOs that are blended in or how long that blend has been used for. There is never an absolute dilution rule, it is you who knows about your level and tolerance. I feel that it is best to start with a higher dilution percentage and increase EO drops over time.

To make sure your EO is safe, make sure that the oils you use are therapeutic grade and do your research on the source and extraction methods used to produce the oils.

Roller Bottle Blending Order

I normally just start with dropping the drops of oil into the **10mL roller bottle**, then adding the carrier oil up until the shoulder of the bottle. Capping the bottle off with the roller and the bottle cap. Instead of shaking the bottle, i like to roll the bottle between my palms first for a minute or 2 for blending, then finishing it off with a few shakes.

NOTE: All recipes in this book is for a 10mL Roller Bottle. If you have a bigger or smaller roller bottle, adjust the number of EO drops based on the size of your bottle.

Roller Bottle Recipes

5 drops Lavender
5 drops Lemon
5 drops Peppermint
----

6 drops Lavender
6 drops Lemon
6 drops Peppermint
----

5 drops Lavender
5 drops Lemon
5 drops Purify
1 drops Frankincense
----

2 drops Oregano
4 drops Lemon
3 drops Protective Blend
----

10 drops Basil
5 drops Lavender
3 drops Lemongrass
2 drops Peppermint
----

3 drops Lavender
3 drops Lemon
3 drops Peppermint
----

4 drops Lavender
3 drops Lemon

3 drops Peppermint

----

4 drops Oregano
8 drops Lemon
6 drops Protective Blend

----

4 drops Oregano
6 drops Lemon
5 drops On Guard
5 drops Melaleuca

----

4 drops Frankincense
4 drops Lemon
4 drops Melaleuca Tea Tree
4 drops Protective Blend

----

2 drops Oregano
2 drops Melaleuca
2 drops Lemon
2 drops Frankincense
2 drops Cinnamon

----

3 drops Orange
3 drops Lemon
3 drops Thieves
3 drops Frankincense

----

8 drops Respiratory Blend
5 drops Eucalyptus
4 drops Frankincense
----

6 drop Cardamom
6 drop Frankincense
----

2 drops Oregano
2 drops Tea Tree
2 drops Lemon
2 drops Frankincense
2 drops Cinnamon
----

4 drops Peppermint
2 drops Eucalyptus
2 drops Lemon
2 drops Rosemary
----

2 drops Lemon
6 drops Lavender
2 drops Peppermint
----

4 drops Peace & Calming
3 drops Lavender

3 drops Frankincense

Bonus Recipes

DIY Essential Oil Allergy Remedy

10 ml Bottle
3 drops peppermint
2 drops lavender
2 drops lemon or eucalyptus
Carrier oil

Spring Blend

10 drops Peppermint
10 drops Lavender
10 drops Lemon
Amber dropper bottle

Basil Eucalyptus Blend

10 drops Basil
10 drops Eucalyptus
10 drops Peppermint
Amber dropper bottle

Citrus Grass Blend

15 drops Bergamot
15 drops Lemongrass
Amber dropper bottle

General Use Allergy Blend

60 drops Bergamot
40 drops Lavender
40 drops Juniper
20 drops Peppermint
10 ml Glass Dropper Bottle

Allergy Blend Air Spray

75 drops of your Allergy Blend Essential Oil
4 Oz Glass Spray Bottle
1 Tsp Vodka
1/2 cup Distilled or Filtered Water

Allergy Blend Hand/Foot/Sitz Bath

1 Tsp Milk
4-6 drops Allergy blend (in a non-reactive
bowl)
Hot water/Warm Water

Allergy Blend Massage Oil

4 tsp Grapeseed or Sweet Almond oil
8 drops Allergy Blend

Inhale

Essential Oil Inhalers are the most convenient way to enjoy Essential Oils Anywhere and Whenever.

Essential Oil Inhalers give you quick and easy access to the vast therapeutic benefits of essential oils.

Blending Essential Oils in an Inhaler
Some Tidbits You Need To Know

EO Inhalers or aroma sticks are compact tubes, with a cotton wick inside and a protective cover, to lock the aroma within.

Your preferred blend of essential oils is absorbed by the cotton wick, and safely enclosed in a tube that fits inside of the cover. The cover is easily removed for access to the tube to breathe in the aroma. Usually lasts about 3 months, depending on the oil blend used.

I absolutely love these because they encourage me to take a moment during super stressful moments, and just breathe.

It is in times of stress when our breathing patterns often change and taking deep breaths promote a feeling of calm and inner peace. Breath work combined with visualization plus a relaxing inhaler, can offer relief to symptoms of stress and help your body to come back to the state of homeostasis.

Aroma Sticks can be carried in your tiny purse, even compact enough to fit in your pocket. You can enjoy your favorite EOs anywhere and you can use them with discretion.

I love diffusing, and do all the time but not everyone in my space may enjoy the scents I enjoy or they may not benefit from the therapeutic benefits of the EOs I am diffusing - so the inhaler is one way to not only enjoy my choice of blends but to keep in personal not affecting everyone else around me.

Inhalers not only benefits me but also keep those around me safe in case the oils I want to blend may pose a risk to those around me who may have a health issue not advised to be exposed to my choice EOs/

When making Aroma Sticks, You may use your chosen EOs at 100% Concentration.

Inhaler Basic Guidelines

Breathe in slow and deep to absorb the EO molecules directly into your olfactory system.

Inhalers are super easy to use. You just remove the cap and inhale from the inhaler tube, count 1 to 5 slowly as you inhale. The EO molecules get drawn into our bloodstream through our nasal cavity and gets delivered throughout our entire body.

Simple to use, easy to cary, portable and compact. You never have to be without your favorite blends, ever.

Inhaler Blending Basics

Inhalers are super easy and simple to make.

All you need is an inhaler set which consist of the following:

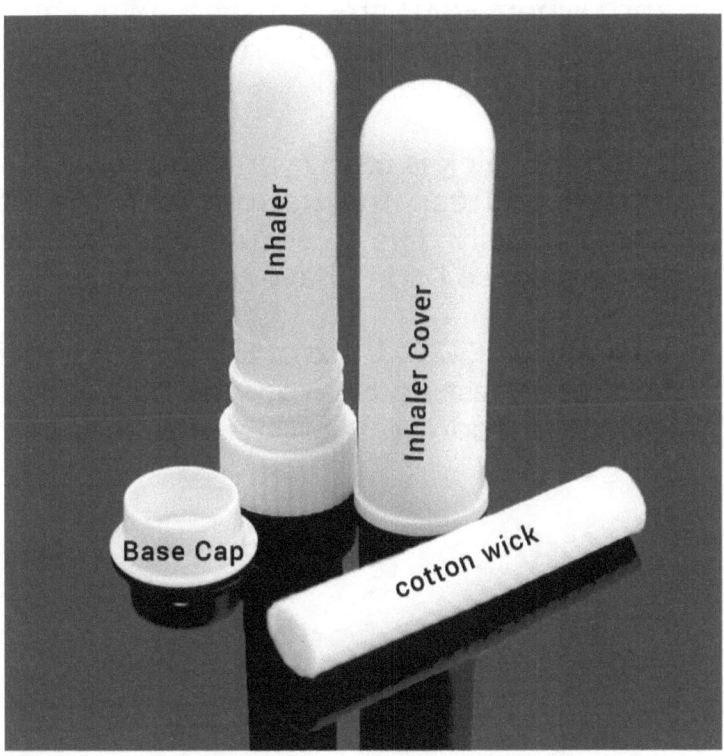

Inhaler, Inhaler Cover, Base Cap and Cotton Wick.

You will need your Essential Oils.

I like to use a pipette for precision and a small petri dish so I can see the oil.

Blending is super easy, just combine the drops and swirl it around in the petri dish and when you are satisfied you can go ahead and drop the cotton wick to absorb all the oil in the dish.

Once the wick is ready you can drop it in the inhaler and cap the bottom with the Base Cap. I usually like to secure the cover with the inhaler so I don't have to do it later.

I usually us 15-20 drops of EO total in a recipe and it can last up to 3 months. Some recipes will need more but on average it is in this range.

Inhaler Recipes

7 drops Eucalyptus
5 drops Tea Tree
5 drops Lemongrass
3 drops Lemon

----

5 drops Cedarwood
5 drops Tea Tree
5 drops Lavender

----

4 drops Frankincense
6 drops Vetiver
5 drops Chamomile

----

4 drops Oregano
2 drops Clove
2 drops Lemon
2 drops Eucalyptus
2 drops Rosemary
4 drops Frankincense

----

3 drops Oregano
3 drops Tea tree
3 drops Lemon
3 drops Frankincense
3 drops Cinnamon leaf

----

5 drops Pine or Cedarwood
5 drops Lavender
4 drops Eucalyptus
1 drop Lemon

----

4 drops Peppermint
4 drops Eucalyptus
2 drops Lavender
2 drops Lemon
3 drops Rosemary

4-6 drops Rosemary
6-8 drops Peppermint
4-6 drops Eucalyptus

----

8 drops Rosemary
5 drops Thyme
2 drop Peppermint

----

5 drops Lavender
5 drops Peppermint
5 drops Lemon

----

10 drops of Rosemary
4 drops of Oregano
2 drops of Peppermint

----

5 drops Eucalyptus
5 drops Peppermint
5 drops Lemon

----

9 drops of Rosemary
3 drop of Pine
3 drops of Peppermint
----

5 drops Cedarwood
5 drops Lavender
5 drops Tea Tree

----

4 drops Peppermint
4 drops Lavender
4 drops Eucalyptus
2 drop Lemon
2 drops Rosemary

----

3 drops Oregano
3 drops Tea tree
3 drops Lemon
3 drops Frankincense
3 drops Cinnamon leaf

----

5 drops Black Pepper
5 drops Frankincense
5 drops Black Spruce

----

5 drops Cypress
5 drops Eucalyptus
5 drops Tea Tree

----

3 drops Eucalyptus
3 drops Thyme
3 drops Peppermint
3 drops Basil
3 drops Rosemary

----

5 drops of Lemon
5 drops of Lavender
5 drops of Peppermint

----

3 drops of Oregano
3 drops of Tea Tree
3 drops of Lemon
3 drops of Frankincense
3 drops of Cinnamon

----

9 drops of Lime
5 drops of Black Spruce
3 drops of Lavender
1 drop of Peppermint

----

10 drop of Black Spruce
6 drops of Lime

XX

Book Ordering

To order your copy / copies of
Essential Oils for Allergies

please visit: **EOrecipes.net**

You can also check out other titles available.

Bulk Pricing and
Affiliate Programs Available

www.ingramcontent.com/pod-product-compliance
Lightning Source LLC
Chambersburg PA
CBHW061216280526
45784CB00006B/2502